The Pharmacy Technician's Pocket Drug Reference

The Pharmacy Technician's Pocket Drug Reference

5th Edition

Joyce A. Generali, BPharm, MS, FASHP
Director, Drug Information Center
University of Kansas Medical Center
Kansas City, Kansas
Clinical Professor
University of Kansas School of Pharmacy
Lawrence, Kansas

American Pharmacists Association®
Improving medication use. Advancing patient care.
APhA
Washington, D.C.

Editor: Nancy Tarleton Landis
Layout and Graphics: Michele Danoff
Cover Design: Scott Neitzke, APhA Creative Services

© 2009 by the American Pharmacists Association
Published by the American Pharmacists Association,
1100 15th Street, N.W., Suite 400, Washington, DC 20005-1707
www.pharmacist.com

APhA was founded in 1852 as the American Pharmaceutical Association.

To comment on this book via e-mail, send your message to the publisher at
aphabooks@aphanet.org.

Library of Congress Cataloging-in-Publication Data

Generali, Joyce A.
  The pharmacy technician's pocket drug reference / Joyce A. Generali.
— 5th ed.
      p. ; cm.
  Includes index.
  ISBN 978-1-58212-123-9
  1. Pharmacy technicians--Handbooks, manuals, etc. 2.
Drugs--Handbooks, manuals, etc. I. American Pharmacists Association.
II. Title.
  [DNLM: 1. Pharmaceutical Preparations—administration & dosage—
Handbooks. 2. Pharmacists' Aides—Handbooks. QV 735 G326p 2009]

    RS122.95.G464 2009
    615'.1--dc22

                                  2008043654

How to Order This Book

Online: www.pharmacist.com

By phone: 800-878-0729 (770-280-0085 from outside the United States).

VISA®, MasterCard®, and American Express® cards accepted

CONTENTS

Because the Food and Drug Administration (FDA) approves approximately 20 to 30 new chemical entities annually, keeping current with new drug products is a continuing concern for pharmacy technicians as well as pharmacists. *The Pharmacy Technician's Pocket Drug Reference* is the first drug information reference designed especially to help pharmacy technicians quickly identify drug products, their uses, and their dosage forms. The drugs included are categorized by generic names, trade names, therapeutic drug classes, general FDA-approved therapeutic uses, and commercially available dosage forms.

Kept concise for quick and easy access, the book can be used at work or during study for examination. When more in-depth drug information is required, referral to other drug information resources and consultation with the supervising pharmacist are always recommended.

Although several brand names are listed for most generic drugs, please note that this is for identification purposes only and does not infer or imply therapeutic or generic equivalency. In addition, all dosage forms may not be available for every trade name listed.

Special care has been taken to include the top 200 most commonly prescribed drugs. In addition, most drugs marketed since 1997 have been included in an attempt to create a resource that is useful in the practice setting.

Note that the information on most injectable formulations is presented in final dose amounts of the container (e.g., syringe, vial, ampul) and not as the concentration of the drug. Amounts provided for injectable formulations are not to be construed as appropriate doses. Some amounts are larger than typical doses because the container is a multidose vial. This resource is not intended as a dosing guide; an appropriate resource should be used in making patient care decisions.

I hope this is a useful addition to your library and optimizes the efficient and safe practice of pharmacy.

Joyce A. Generali, BPharm, MS, FASHP
October 2008

ABACAVIR
a BAK a veer
TRADE NAME(S):
Ziagen
THERAPEUTIC CLASS:
Antiviral
GENERAL USES:
HIV infection
DOSAGE FORMS:
Tablets: 300 mg; Solution:
20 mg/mL

ABACAVIR/LAMIVUDINE
a BAK aveer/la MI vyoo
deen
TRADE NAME(S):
Epzicom
THERAPEUTIC CLASS:
Antiviral
GENERAL USES:
HIV infection
DOSAGE FORMS:
Tablets: 600 mg/300 mg

**ABACAVIR/LAMIVUDINE/
ZIDOVUDINE**
a BAK a veer/la MI vyoo
deen/zye DOE vyoo deen
TRADE NAME(S):
Trizivir
THERAPEUTIC CLASS:
Antiviral
GENERAL USES:
HIV infection
DOSAGE FORMS:
Tablets: 300 mg/150 mg/
300 mg

ABATACEPT
ab a TA sept
TRADE NAME(S):
Orencia
THERAPEUTIC CLASS:
Antirheumatic
GENERAL USES:
Rheumatoid arthritis
DOSAGE FORMS:
Injection: 250 mg

**ACAMPROSATE
CALCIUM**
ay CAM pro sate
TRADE NAME(S):
Campral
THERAPEUTIC CLASS:
Antialcoholism agent
GENERAL USES:
Alcohol dependence
DOSAGE FORMS:
Delayed-release tablets:
333 mg

ACARBOSE
AY car bose
TRADE NAME(S):
Precose
THERAPEUTIC CLASS:
Antidiabetic
GENERAL USES:
Diabetes (type 2)
DOSAGE FORMS:
Tablets: 25 mg, 50 mg,
100 mg

ACEBUTOLOL
a se BYOO toe lole

TRADE NAME(S):
Sectral

THERAPEUTIC CLASS:
Antihypertensive,
antiarrhythmic

GENERAL USES:
Hypertension, arrhythmias

DOSAGE FORMS:
Capsules: 200 mg,
400 mg

ACETAMINOPHEN
a seet a MIN oh fen

TRADE NAME(S):
Tylenol, Tempra, Aceta,
many others

THERAPEUTIC CLASS:
Analgesic,
antipyretic

GENERAL USES:
Pain, fever

DOSAGE FORMS:
Tablets: 160 mg, 325 mg,
500 mg, 650 mg;
Chewable tablets: 80 mg;
Caplets: 160 mg, 500 mg,
650 mg; Capsules:
325 mg, 500 mg; Drops:
80 mg/0.8 mL; Also Elixir,
Liquid, and Solution

ACETOHEXAMIDE
a set oh HEKS a mide

TRADE NAME(S):
Dymelor

THERAPEUTIC CLASS:
Antidiabetic

GENERAL USES:
Diabetes (type 2)

DOSAGE FORMS:
Tablets: 250 mg, 500 mg

ACETYLCYSTEINE
a se teel SIS teen

TRADE NAME(S):
Acetadote, Mucomyst

THERAPEUTIC CLASS:
Antidote

GENERAL USES:
Acetaminophen overdose

DOSAGE FORMS:
Injection: 20%;
Solution: 10%, 20%

ACITRETIN
a si TRE tin

TRADE NAME(S):
Soriatane

THERAPEUTIC CLASS:
Retinoid

GENERAL USES:
Psoriasis

DOSAGE FORMS:
Capsules: 10 mg, 25 mg

ACYCLOVIR
ay SYE kloe veer

TRADE NAME(S):
Zovirax

THERAPEUTIC CLASS:
Antiviral

GENERAL USES:
Herpes, shingles,
chickenpox

DOSAGE FORMS:
Tablets: 400 mg,
800 mg; Capsules:
200 mg; Suspension:
200 mg/5 mL; Cream and
Ointment: 5%; Injection:
500 mg, 1 g

ADALIMUMAB
a da LIM yoo mab
TRADE NAME(S):
Humira
THERAPEUTIC CLASS:
Monoclonal antibody
GENERAL USES:
Rheumatoid arthritis,
ankylosing spondylitis
DOSAGE FORMS:
Injection: 40 mg

ADAPALENE
a DAP a leen
TRADE NAME(S):
Differin
THERAPEUTIC CLASS:
Retinoid (topical)
GENERAL USES:
Acne vulgaris
DOSAGE FORMS:
Topical gel, Cream,
Solution: 0.1%, 0.3%

ADEFOVIR DIPIVOXIL
a DEF o veer dye pi
VOKS il
TRADE NAME(S):
Hepsera

THERAPEUTIC CLASS:
Antiviral
GENERAL USES:
Chronic hepatitis B
DOSAGE FORMS:
Tablets: 10 mg

AGALSIDASE BETA
ay GAL si days
TRADE NAME(S):
Fabrazyme
THERAPEUTIC CLASS:
Enzyme
GENERAL USES:
Fabry's disease
DOSAGE FORMS:
Injection: 5 mg, 35 mg

ALBUTEROL
al BYOO ter ole
TRADE NAME(S):
Proventil, Proventil HFA,
Ventolin HFA
THERAPEUTIC CLASS:
Bronchodilator
GENERAL USES:
Bronchospasm
DOSAGE FORMS:
Tablets: 2 mg, 4 mg;
Extended-release tablets:
4 mg, 8 mg; Syrup: 2 mg/
5 mL; Aerosol: 90 mcg/
inhalation; Inhalation
solution: 0.021%,
0.042%, 0.083%, 0.5%

ALCLOMETASONE
al kloe MET a sone
TRADE NAME(S):
Aclovate
THERAPEUTIC CLASS:
Corticosteroid
GENERAL USES:
Various skin conditions
DOSAGE FORMS:
Ointment and Cream:
0.05%

ALEFACEPT
a LE fa sept
TRADE NAME(S):
Amevive
THERAPEUTIC CLASS:
Monoclonal antibody
GENERAL USES:
Plaque psoriasis
DOSAGE FORMS:
Injection: 15 mg

ALEMTUZUMAB
ay lem TU zoo mab
TRADE NAME(S):
Campath
THERAPEUTIC CLASS:
Monoclonal antibody
GENERAL USES:
Refractory leukemia
DOSAGE FORMS:
Injection: 30 mg

ALENDRONATE
a LEN droe nate
TRADE NAME(S):
Fosamax

THERAPEUTIC CLASS:
Bisphosphonate
GENERAL USES:
Osteoporosis, Paget's
disease
DOSAGE FORMS:
Tablets: 5 mg, 10 mg,
35 mg, 40 mg, 70 mg;
Oral solution: 70 mg/
75 mL

**ALENDRONATE/
CHOLECALCIFEROL**
a LEN droe nate/kole eh kal
SI fer ole
TRADE NAME(S):
Fosamax Plus D
THERAPEUTIC CLASS:
Bisphosphonate/
Vitamin
GENERAL USES:
Osteoporosis
DOSAGE FORMS:
Tablets: 70 mg/
2800 international units
(IU), 70 mg/5600 IU

ALFUZOSIN
al FYOO zoe sin
TRADE NAME(S):
Uroxatral
THERAPEUTIC CLASS:
Urologic agent
GENERAL USES:
BPH
DOSAGE FORMS:
Extended-release tablets:
10 mg

ALGLUCOSIDASE ALFA
al gloo KOSE i dase AL fa

TRADE NAME(S):
Myozyme

THERAPEUTIC CLASS:
Enzyme

GENERAL USES:
Pompe disease

DOSAGE FORMS:
Injection: 50 mg

ALISKIREN
a lis KYE ren

TRADE NAME(S):
Tekturna

THERAPEUTIC CLASS:
Antihypertensive

GENERAL USES:
Hypertension

DOSAGE FORMS:
Tablets: 150 mg, 300 mg

ALISKIREN/HCTZ
a lis KYE ren/hye droe klor oh THYE a zide

TRADE NAME(S):
Tekturna HCT

THERAPEUTIC CLASS:
Antihypertensive/ diuretic

GENERAL USES:
Hypertension

DOSAGE FORMS:
Tablets: 150 mg/12.5 mg, 150 mg/25 mg, 300 mg/ 12.5 mg, 300 mg/25 mg

ALITRETINOIN
a li TRET i noyn

TRADE NAME(S):
Panretin

THERAPEUTIC CLASS:
Retinoid (topical)

GENERAL USES:
Kaposi's sarcoma cutaneous lesions

DOSAGE FORMS:
Topical gel: 0.1%

ALLOPURINOL
al oh PURE i nole

TRADE NAME(S):
Zyloprim

THERAPEUTIC CLASS:
Gout agent

GENERAL USES:
Gout, increased uric acid conditions, calcium stones

DOSAGE FORMS:
Tablets: 100 mg, 300 mg; Injection: 500 mg

ALMOTRIPTAN
al moh TRIP tan

TRADE NAME(S):
Axert

THERAPEUTIC CLASS:
Antimigraine agent

GENERAL USES:
Migraine treatment

DOSAGE FORMS:
Tablets: 6.25 mg, 12.5 mg

ALOSETRON
al OH seh trahn
TRADE NAME(S):
Lotronex
THERAPEUTIC CLASS:
GI agent
GENERAL USES:
Irritable bowel syndrome
(women)
DOSAGE FORMS:
Tablets: 0.5 mg, 1 mg

ALPRAZOLAM
al PRAY zoe lam
TRADE NAME(S):
Xanax, Xanax XR,
Alprazolam Intensol,
Niravam
THERAPEUTIC CLASS:
Antianxiety agent
GENERAL USES:
Anxiety, panic disorder
DOSAGE FORMS:
Tablets: 0.25 mg,
0.5 mg, 1 mg, 2 mg;
Solution: 1 mg/mL;
Extended-release tablets:
0.5 mg, 1 mg, 2 mg, 3 mg;
Orally disintegrating
tablets: 0.25 mg, 0.5 mg,
1 mg, 2 mg

ALTEPLASE
AL te plase
TRADE NAME(S):
Activase,
Cath-Flo Activase

THERAPEUTIC CLASS:
Thrombolytic agent
GENERAL USES:
Dissolves blood clots in
MI, stroke, pulmonary
embolism, catheter
occlusion
DOSAGE FORMS:
Injection: 2 mg, 50 mg,
100 mg

ALVIMOPAN
al vi MOE pan
TRADE NAME(S):
Entereg
THERAPEUTIC CLASS:
GI agent
GENERAL USES:
Postoperative ileus
DOSAGE FORMS:
Capsules: 12 mg

AMANTADINE
a MAN ta deen
TRADE NAME(S):
Symmetrel
THERAPEUTIC CLASS:
Antiparkinson agent
GENERAL USES:
Parkinson's disease, drug-
induced extrapyramidal
disorders
DOSAGE FORMS:
Tablets and Capsules:
100 mg; Syrup: 50 mg/
5 mL

AMBRISENTAN
am bree SEN tan
TRADE NAME(S):
Letairis
THERAPEUTIC CLASS:
Antihypertensive
GENERAL USES:
Pulmonary hypertension
DOSAGE FORMS:
Tablets: 5 mg, 10 mg

AMCINONIDE
am SIN oh nide
TRADE NAME(S):
Cyclocort
THERAPEUTIC CLASS:
Corticosteroid (topical)
GENERAL USES:
Various skin conditions
DOSAGE FORMS:
Ointment, Cream, and
Lotion: 0.1%

AMIKACIN
am i KAY sin
TRADE NAME(S):
Amikin
THERAPEUTIC CLASS:
Anti-infective
GENERAL USES:
Bacterial infections
DOSAGE FORMS:
Injection: 100 mg,
200 mg, 500 mg, 1 g

AMILORIDE
a MIL oh ride

TRADE NAME(S):
Midamor
THERAPEUTIC CLASS:
Diuretic
GENERAL USES:
CHF-related edema,
hypertension
DOSAGE FORMS:
Tablets: 5 mg

AMINOCAPROIC ACID
a mee noe ka PROE ik
TRADE NAME(S):
Amicar
THERAPEUTIC CLASS:
Hemostatic
GENERAL USES:
Excessive bleeding
DOSAGE FORMS:
Tablets: 500 mg; Syrup:
250 mg/mL

**AMINOLEVULINIC
ACID**
a MEE noh lev yoo lin ik
TRADE NAME(S):
Levulan Kerastick
THERAPEUTIC CLASS:
Skin agent (topical)
GENERAL USES:
Precancerous skin lesions
on face or scalp
DOSAGE FORMS:
Topical solution: 20%

AMINOPHYLLINE
am in OFF i lin

Trade Name(s)
Phyllocontin

Therapeutic Class:
Bronchodilator

General Uses:
Asthma

Dosage Forms:
(equivalent amount of theophylline):
Tablets: 100 mg (79 mg), 200 mg (158 mg);
Controlled-release tablets: 225 mg (178 mg);
Oral liquid: 105 mg/5 mL (90 mg/5 mL);
Injection: 250 mg (197 mg), 500 mg (394 mg)

AMIODARONE
a MEE oh da rone

Trade Name(s):
Cordarone, Cordarone IV, Pacerone

Therapeutic Class:
Antiarrhythmic

General Uses:
Ventricular arrhythmias and fibrillation

Dosage Forms:
Tablets: 100 mg, 200 mg, 300 mg, 400 mg;
Injection: 150 mg

AMITRIPTYLINE
a mee TRIP ti leen

Trade Name(s):
Elavil

Therapeutic Class:
Antidepressant

General Uses:
Depression

Dosage Forms:
Tablets: 10 mg, 25 mg, 50 mg, 75 mg, 100 mg, 150 mg

AMLODIPINE
am LOE di peen

Trade Name(s):
Norvasc

Therapeutic Class:
Antihypertensive, antianginal

General Uses:
Hypertension, angina

Dosage Forms:
Tablets: 2.5 mg, 5 mg, 10 mg

AMLODIPINE/ ATORVASTATIN
am LOE di peen/a TORE va sta tin

Trade Name(s):
Caduet

Therapeutic Class:
Antihypertensive/ antilipemic

General Uses:
Hypertension, angina, lipid disorders

DOSAGE FORMS:
Tablets: 2.5 mg/10 mg,
5 mg/10 mg, 10 mg/
10 mg, 2.5 mg/20 mg,
5 mg/20 mg, 10 mg/
20 mg, 2.5 mg/40 mg,
5 mg/40 mg, 10 mg/
40 mg, 5 mg/80 mg,
10 mg/80 mg

AMLODIPINE/ BENAZEPRIL
am LOE di peen/ben AY ze pril
TRADE NAME(S):
Lotrel
THERAPEUTIC CLASS:
Antihypertensive/
diuretic
GENERAL USES:
CHF, hypertension
DOSAGE FORMS:
Tablets: 2.5 mg/10 mg,
5 mg/10 mg, 5 mg/20 mg,
5 mg/40 mg, 10 mg/
20 mg, 10 mg/40 mg

AMLODIPINE/ OLMESARTAN
am LOE di peen/ole me
SAR tan
TRADE NAME(S):
Azor
THERAPEUTIC CLASS:
Antihypertensive
GENERAL USES:
Hypertension
DOSAGE FORMS:
Tablets: 5 mg/20 mg,
5 mg/40 mg, 10 mg/
20 mg, 10 mg/40 mg

AMLODIPINE/ VALSARTAN
am LOE di peen/val
SAR tan
TRADE NAME(S):
Exforge
THERAPEUTIC CLASS:
Antihypertensive
GENERAL USES:
Hypertension
DOSAGE FORMS:
Tablets: 5 mg/160 mg,
5 mg/320 mg, 10 mg/
160 mg, 10 mg/320 mg

AMOXAPINE
a MOKS a peen
TRADE NAME(S):
Asendin
THERAPEUTIC CLASS:
Antidepressant
GENERAL USES:
Depression
DOSAGE FORMS:
Tablets: 25 mg, 50 mg,
100 mg, 150 mg

AMOXICILLIN
a moks i SIL in
TRADE NAME(S):
Amoxil, Moxatag, Trimox,
Wymox
THERAPEUTIC CLASS:
Anti-infective

GENERAL USES:
Bacterial infections
DOSAGE FORMS:
Chewable tablets: 125 mg, 200 mg, 250 mg, 400 mg; Tablets: 500 mg; 875 mg; Extended-release tablets: 775 mg; Capsules: 250 mg, 500 mg; Suspension: 50 mg/mL, 125 mg/5 mL, 200 mg/ 5 mL, 250 mg/5 mL, 400 mg/5 mL; Tablets for oral suspension: 200 mg, 400 mg

AMOXICILLIN/ CLAVULANATE
a moks i SIL in/klav yoo LAN ate
TRADE NAME(S):
Augmentin, Augmentin ES, Augmentin XR
THERAPEUTIC CLASS:
Anti-infective
GENERAL USES:
Bacterial infections
DOSAGE FORMS:
Tablets: 250 mg/125 mg, 500 mg/125 mg, 875 mg/ 125 mg; Chewable tablets and Suspension (per 5 mL): 125 mg/31.25 mg, 200 mg/28.5 mg, 250 mg/62.5 mg, 400 mg/57 mg; High-

dose suspension: 600 mg/42.9 mg (per 5 mL); Extended-release tablets: 1000 mg/62.5 mg

AMPHOTERICIN B (ORAL)
am foe TER i sin
TRADE NAME(S):
Fungizone
THERAPEUTIC CLASS:
Antifungal
GENERAL USES:
Oral fungal infection (candidiasis)
DOSAGE FORMS:
Suspension: 100 mg/ mL; Cream, Lotion, and Ointment: 3%

AMPHOTERICIN B DESOXYCHOLATE (NONLIPID BASED)
am foe TER i sin bee des oks ee KOE late
TRADE NAME(S):
Fungizone, Amphocin
THERAPEUTIC CLASS:
Antifungal
GENERAL USES:
Systemic fungal infections
DOSAGE FORMS:
Injection: 50 mg

AMPHOTERICIN B, LIPID BASED
am foe TER i sin

TRADE NAME(S):
Abelcet, Amphotec,
AmBisome
THERAPEUTIC CLASS:
Antifungal
GENERAL USES:
Systemic fungal
infections
DOSAGE FORMS:
Injection: 50 mg, 100 mg

AMPICILLIN
am pi SIL in
TRADE NAME(S):
Principen, Omnipen,
Totacillin
THERAPEUTIC CLASS:
Anti-infective
GENERAL USES:
Bacterial infections
DOSAGE FORMS:
Capsules: 250 mg,
500 mg; Suspension:
125 mg/5 mL, 250 mg/
5 mL; Injection: 125 mg,
250 mg, 500 mg, 1 g, 2 g,
10 g

AMPICILLIN SODIUM/ SULBACTAM SODIUM
am pi SIL in/SUL bak tam
TRADE NAME(S):
Unasyn
THERAPEUTIC CLASS:
Anti-infective
GENERAL USES:
Bacterial infections

DOSAGE FORMS:
Injection: 1 g/0.5 g,
2 g/1 g, 10 g/5 g

ANAGRELIDE
an AG gre lide
TRADE NAME(S):
Agrylin
THERAPEUTIC CLASS:
Antiplatelet agent
GENERAL USES:
Essential
thrombocytopenia
DOSAGE FORMS:
Capsules: 0.5 mg,
1 mg

ANAKINRA
an a KIN ra
TRADE NAME(S):
Kineret
THERAPEUTIC CLASS:
Biological
GENERAL USES:
Rheumatoid
arthritis
DOSAGE FORMS:
Injection: 100 mg

ANASTROZOLE
an AS troe zole
TRADE NAME(S):
Arimidex
THERAPEUTIC CLASS:
Antineoplastic
GENERAL USES:
Breast cancer

DOSAGE FORMS:
Tablets: 1 mg

ANIDULAFUNGIN
ay nid yoo la FUN jin
TRADE NAME(S):
Eraxis
THERAPEUTIC CLASS:
Antifungal
GENERAL USES:
Candidemia, candidiasis
DOSAGE FORMS:
Injection: 50 mg, 100 mg

ANTHRALIN
AN thra lin
TRADE NAME(S):
Anthra-Derm,
Drithocreme
THERAPEUTIC CLASS:
Antipsoriatic (topical)
GENERAL USES:
Psoriasis
DOSAGE FORMS:
Ointment and Cream:
0.1%, 0.25%, 0.4%,
0.5%, 1%; Cream: 0.2%

**ANTIHEMOPHILIC FACTOR
(RECOMBINANT)**
AN tee hee moe FIL ik
TRADE NAME(S):
Xyntha
THERAPEUTIC CLASS:
Hematological agent
GENERAL USES:
Prevent/control
hemorrhage

DOSAGE FORMS:
Injection: 250 international
units (IU), 500 IU,
1000 IU, 2000 IU

APOMORPHINE
a poe MOR feen
TRADE NAME(S):
Apokyn
THERAPEUTIC CLASS:
Dopamine agonist
GENERAL USES:
Parkinson's disease
DOSAGE FORMS:
Injection: 20 mg,
30 mg

APRACLONIDINE
a pra KLOE ni deen
TRADE NAME(S):
Iopidine
THERAPEUTIC CLASS:
Ocular agent
GENERAL USES:
Decrease intraocular
pressure
DOSAGE FORMS:
Ophthalmic solution:
0.5%, 1%

APREPITANT
ap RE pi tant
TRADE NAME(S):
Emend
THERAPEUTIC CLASS:
Antiemetic
GENERAL USES:
Chemotherapy-induced

or postoperative nausea/
vomiting
DOSAGE FORMS:
Capsules: 40 mg, 80 mg,
125 mg

ARFORMOTEROL
ar for MOE ter ol
TRADE NAME(S):
Brovana
THERAPEUTIC CLASS:
Bronchodilator
GENERAL USES:
COPD
DOSAGE FORMS:
Inhalation solution:
15 mcg/2 mL

ARGATROBAN
ar GA troh ban
TRADE NAME(S):
Acova
THERAPEUTIC CLASS:
Anticoagulant
GENERAL USES:
Anticoagulation in
hemodialysis or PCI
DOSAGE FORMS:
Injection: 250 mg

ARIPIPRAZOLE
ay ri PIP ray zole
TRADE NAME(S):
Abilify, Abilify Discmelt
THERAPEUTIC CLASS:
Antipsychotic
GENERAL USES:
Psychotic disorders

DOSAGE FORMS:
Tablets: 5 mg, 10 mg,
15 mg, 20 mg, 30 mg;
Oral solution: 1 mg/1 mL;
Orally disintegrating
tablets: 10 mg, 15 mg,
20 mg, 30 mg; Injection:
7.5 mg

ARMODAFINIL
ar moe DAF in il
TRADE NAME(S):
Nuvigil
THERAPEUTIC CLASS:
Stimulant
GENERAL USES:
Excessive sleepiness,
narcolepsy, obstructive
sleep apnea
DOSAGE FORMS:
Tablets: 50 mg, 150 mg,
250 mg

ARSENIC TRIOXIDE
AR se nik tri OKS id
TRADE NAME(S):
Trisenox
THERAPEUTIC CLASS:
Antineoplastic
GENERAL USES:
Acute promyelocytic
leukemia
DOSAGE FORMS:
Injection: 10 mg

ASPIRIN
AS pir in

TRADE NAME(S):
Empirin, ZORprin, many others

THERAPEUTIC CLASS:
Analgesic, antipyretic, anti-inflammatory

GENERAL USES:
Pain, fever (adults), arthritis

DOSAGE FORMS:
Tablets: 81 mg, 165 mg, 325 mg, 500 mg, 650 mg, 975 mg;
Extended-release tablets: 650 mg, 800 mg

ASPIRIN/ DIPYRIDAMOLE
AS pir in/dye peer ID a mole

TRADE NAME(S):
Aggrenox

THERAPEUTIC CLASS:
Antithrombotic

GENERAL USES:
Reduce stroke risk

DOSAGE FORMS:
Capsules: 25 mg/ 200 mg

ATAZANAVIR SULFATE
at a za NA veer

TRADE NAME(S):
Reyataz

THERAPEUTIC CLASS:
Antiviral

GENERAL USES:
HIV infection

DOSAGE FORMS:
Capsules: 100 mg, 150 mg, 200 mg, 300 mg

ATENOLOL
a TEN oh lole

TRADE NAME(S):
Tenormin

THERAPEUTIC CLASS:
Cardiac agent

GENERAL USES:
Hypertension

DOSAGE FORMS:
Tablets: 25 mg, 50 mg, 100 mg; Injection: 5 mg

ATENOLOL/ CHLORTHALIDONE
a TEN oh lole/klor THAL i done

TRADE NAME(S):
Tenoretic

THERAPEUTIC CLASS:
Antihypertensive/diuretic

GENERAL USES:
Hypertension

DOSAGE FORMS:
Tablets: 100 mg/25 mg, 50 mg/25 mg

ATOMOXETINE
AT oh mox e teen

TRADE NAME(S):
Strattera

THERAPEUTIC CLASS:
Nonstimulant agent

GENERAL USES:
ADHD

DOSAGE FORMS:
  Capsules: 10 mg, 18 mg,
  25 mg, 40 mg, 60 mg,
  80 mg, 100 mg

ATORVASTATIN
a TORE va sta tin
TRADE NAME(S):
  Lipitor
THERAPEUTIC CLASS:
  Antilipemic
GENERAL USES:
  Hyperlipidemia,
  hypertriglyceridemia,
  reduce stroke or MI risk
DOSAGE FORMS:
  Tablets: 10 mg, 20 mg,
  40 mg, 80 mg

ATOVAQUONE/ PROGUANIL
a TOE va kwone/pro
GWA nil
TRADE NAME(S):
  Malarone,
  Malarone-Pediatric
THERAPEUTIC CLASS:
  Antimalarial
GENERAL USES:
  Malaria treatment and
  prevention
DOSAGE FORMS:
  Tablets: 250 mg/100 mg,
  62.5 mg/25 mg

ATROPINE
A troe peen

TRADE NAME(S):
  Isopto Atropine
THERAPEUTIC CLASS:
  Ocular agent
GENERAL USES:
  Pupil dilation
DOSAGE FORMS:
  Ophthalmic solution:
  0.5%, 1%, 2%;
  Ophthalmic ointment: 1%

AURANOFIN
au RANE oh fin
TRADE NAME(S):
  Ridaura
THERAPEUTIC CLASS:
  Antirheumatic agent
GENERAL USES:
  Rheumatoid arthritis
DOSAGE FORMS:
  Capsules: 3 mg

AZACITIDINE
ay za SYE ti deen
TRADE NAME(S):
  Vidaza
THERAPEUTIC CLASS:
  Antineoplastic
GENERAL USES:
  Myelodysplastic
  syndrome
DOSAGE FORMS:
  Injection: 100 mg

AZELASTINE (NASAL)
a ZEL as teen
TRADE NAME(S):
  Astelin

THERAPEUTIC CLASS:
  Antihistamine
GENERAL USES:
  Allergies
DOSAGE FORMS:
  Nasal spray: 137 mcg/spray

AZELASTINE (OCULAR)
a ZEL as teen
TRADE NAME(S):
  Optivar
THERAPEUTIC CLASS:
  Ocular agent
  (antihistamine)
GENERAL USES:
  Allergic conjunctivitis
DOSAGE FORMS:
  Ophthalmic solution:
  0.05%

AZITHROMYCIN
az ith roe MYE sin
TRADE NAME(S):
  Zithromax, Zmax
THERAPEUTIC CLASS:
  Anti-infective
GENERAL USES:
  Bacterial infections
DOSAGE FORMS:
  Tablets: 250 mg, 500 mg,
  600 mg; Suspension:
  100 mg/5 mL, 200 mg/
  5 mL; Injection: 500 mg

AZITHROMYCIN
(OCULAR)
az ith roe MYE sin

TRADE NAME(S):
  AzaSite
THERAPEUTIC CLASS:
  Anti-infective (ocular)
GENERAL USES:
  Bacterial conjunctivitis
DOSAGE FORMS:
  Ophthalmic solution: 1%

AZTREONAM
AZ tree oh nam
TRADE NAME(S):
  Azactam
THERAPEUTIC CLASS:
  Anti-infective
GENERAL USES:
  Bacterial infections
DOSAGE FORMS:
  Injection: 500 mg,
  1 g, 2 g

BACITRACIN
bas i TRAY sin
TRADE NAME(S):
  AK-Tracin
THERAPEUTIC CLASS:
  Ocular agent (anti-
  infective)
GENERAL USES:
  Ocular infections
DOSAGE FORMS:
  Ophthalmic
  ointment:
  500 units/g

BACLOFEN
BAK loe fen

TRADE NAME(S):
Lioresal, Lioresal
Intrathecal

THERAPEUTIC CLASS:
Skeletal muscle relaxant

GENERAL USES:
Spasticity

DOSAGE FORMS:
Tablets: 10 mg, 20 mg;
Injection: 0.05 mg,
0.5 mg, 2 mg

BALSALAZIDE
bal SAL a zide

TRADE NAME(S):
Colazal

THERAPEUTIC CLASS:
GI agent

GENERAL USES:
Ulcerative colitis

DOSAGE FORMS:
Capsules: 750 mg

BECAPLERMIN
be KAP ler min

TRADE NAME(S):
Regranex

THERAPEUTIC CLASS:
Wound healer (topical)

GENERAL USES:
Diabetic neuropathic
ulcers

DOSAGE FORMS:
Topical gel: 0.01%

BECLOMETHASONE
(INHALED)
be kloe METH a sone

TRADE NAME(S):
Vanceril, Beclovent,
Qvar

THERAPEUTIC CLASS:
Corticosteroid (inhaler)

GENERAL USES:
Asthma (chronic)

DOSAGE FORMS:
Inhaler: 40 mcg/
inhalation, 42 mcg/
inhalation, 80 mcg/
inhalation, 84 mcg/
inhalation

BECLOMETHASONE
(NASAL)
be kloe METH a sone

TRADE NAME(S):
Beconase, Vancenase,
Beconase AQ, Vancenase
AQ

THERAPEUTIC CLASS:
Corticosteroid (nasal)

GENERAL USES:
Allergies

DOSAGE FORMS:
Nasal spray: 0.042%,
0.084%

BENAZEPRIL
ben AY ze pril

TRADE NAME(S):
Lotensin

THERAPEUTIC CLASS:
Antihypertensive

GENERAL USES:
Hypertension

DOSAGE FORMS:
Tablets: 5 mg, 10 mg,
20 mg, 40 mg

BENAZEPRIL/HCTZ
ben AY ze pril/hye droe klor
oh THYE a zide
TRADE NAME(S):
Lotensin HCT
THERAPEUTIC CLASS:
Antihypertensive/
diuretic
GENERAL USES:
Hypertension
DOSAGE FORMS:
Tablets: 5 mg/6.25 mg,
10 mg/12.5 mg, 20 mg/
12.5 mg, 20 mg/25 mg

BENDAMUSTINE
ben da MUS teen
TRADE NAME(S):
Treanda
THERAPEUTIC CLASS:
Antineoplastic
GENERAL USES:
Chronic lymphocytic
leukemia
DOSAGE FORMS:
Injection: 100 mg

BENZONATATE
ben ZOE na tate
TRADE NAME(S):
Tessalon Perles
THERAPEUTIC CLASS:
Nonnarcotic cough

suppressant
GENERAL USES:
Relief of cough
DOSAGE FORMS:
Capsules: 100 mg

BENZOYL PEROXIDE
BEN zoyl per OKS ide
TRADE NAME(S):
Benzac, PanOxyl, Persa-
Gel, many others
THERAPEUTIC CLASS:
Anti-infective (topical)
GENERAL USES:
Acne
DOSAGE FORMS:
Liquid, Lotion, Cream,
Gel: 2.5%, 5%, 10%

**BENZOYL PEROXIDE/
CLINDAMYCIN
(TOPICAL)**
BEN zoyl per OKS ide/klin
da MYE sin
TRADE NAME(S):
BenzaClin, Duac
THERAPEUTIC CLASS:
Anti-infective (topical)
GENERAL USES:
Acne
DOSAGE FORMS:
Gel: 5%/1%

BENZTROPINE
BENZ troe peen
TRADE NAME(S):
Cogentin

THERAPEUTIC CLASS:
Antiparkinson agent
GENERAL USES:
Parkinson's disease, drug-induced extrapyramidal disorders
DOSAGE FORMS:
Tablets: 0.5 mg, 1 mg, 2 mg

BEPRIDIL
BE pri dil
TRADE NAME(S):
Vascor
THERAPEUTIC CLASS:
Antianginal
GENERAL USES:
Angina
DOSAGE FORMS:
Tablets: 200 mg, 300 mg, 400 mg

BETAMETHASONE DIPROPRIONATE
bay ta METH a sone
TRADE NAME(S):
Diprosone, Alphatrex, Maxivate
THERAPEUTIC CLASS:
Corticosteroid (topical)
GENERAL USES:
Various skin conditions
DOSAGE FORMS:
Ointment, Cream, and Lotion: 0.05%; Aerosol: 0.1%

BETAMETHASONE VALERATE
bay ta METH a sone
TRADE NAME(S):
Betatrex, Valisone
THERAPEUTIC CLASS:
Corticosteroid (topical)
GENERAL USES:
Various skin conditions
DOSAGE FORMS:
Ointment, Cream, and Lotion: 0.1%; Cream: 0.01%, 0.05%

BETAXOLOL (OCULAR)
be TAKS oh lol
TRADE NAME(S):
Betoptic, Betoptic S
THERAPEUTIC CLASS:
Ocular agent
GENERAL USES:
Glaucoma/ocular hypertension
DOSAGE FORMS:
Ophthalmic solution: 0.5%; Ophthalmic suspension: 0.25%

BETAXOLOL (ORAL)
be TAKS oh lol
TRADE NAME(S):
Kerlone
THERAPEUTIC CLASS:
Antihypertensive

GENERAL USES:
Hypertension
DOSAGE FORMS:
Tablets: 10 mg,
20 mg

BEVACIZUMAB
be va SIZ yoo mab
TRADE NAME(S):
Avastin
THERAPEUTIC CLASS:
Antineoplastic
GENERAL USES:
Metastatic colorectal
cancer
DOSAGE FORMS:
Injection: 100 mg, 400 mg

BEXAROTENE
beks AIR oh teen
TRADE NAME(S):
Targretin
THERAPEUTIC CLASS:
Antineoplastic
GENERAL USES:
T-cell lymphoma
DOSAGE FORMS:
Capsules: 75 mg;
Gel: 1%

BICALUTAMIDE
bye ka LOO ta mide
TRADE NAME(S):
Casodex
THERAPEUTIC CLASS:
Antiandrogen

antineoplastic
GENERAL USES:
Prostate cancer
DOSAGE FORMS:
Tablets: 50 mg

BIMATOPROST
bi MAT oh prost
TRADE NAME(S):
Lumigan
THERAPEUTIC CLASS:
Ocular agent
GENERAL USES:
Ocular hypertension,
open-angle glaucoma
DOSAGE FORMS:
Ophthalmic solution: 0.03%

BIPERIDEN
bye PER i den
TRADE NAME(S):
Akineton
THERAPEUTIC CLASS:
Antiparkinson agent
GENERAL USES:
Parkinson's disease, drug-
induced extrapyramidal
disorders
DOSAGE FORMS:
Tablets: 2 mg

**BISMUTH SUBCITRATE
POTASSIUM/
METRONIDAZOLE/
TETRACYCLINE**
BIZ muth/me troe NI da
zole/tet ra SYE kleen

TRADE NAME(S):
Pylera

THERAPEUTIC CLASS:
Anti-infective

GENERAL USES:
Helicobacter pylori
infection-related ulcers

DOSAGE FORMS:
Capsules: 140 mg/
125 mg/125 mg

BISOPROLOL
bis OH proe lol

TRADE NAME(S):
Zebeta

THERAPEUTIC CLASS:
Antihypertensive

GENERAL USES:
Hypertension

DOSAGE FORMS:
Tablets: 5 mg, 10 mg

BISOPROLOL/HCTZ
bis OH proe lol/hye droe klor
oh THYE a zide

TRADE NAME(S):
Ziac

THERAPEUTIC CLASS:
Antihypertensive/
diuretic

GENERAL USES:
Hypertension

DOSAGE FORMS:
Tablets: 2.5 mg/6.25 mg,
5 mg/6.25 mg, 10 mg/
6.25 mg

BITOLTEROL
bye TOLE ter ole

TRADE NAME(S):
Tornalate

THERAPEUTIC CLASS:
Bronchodilator

GENERAL USES:
Bronchospasm/asthma

DOSAGE FORMS:
Inhalation solution: 0.2%;
Aerosol: 0.8%

BIVALIRUDIN
bye VAL i roo din

TRADE NAME(S):
Angiomax

THERAPEUTIC CLASS:
Anticoagulant

GENERAL USES:
Prevention of clotting in
angina/PTCA

DOSAGE FORMS:
Injection: 250 mg

BORTEZOMIB
bore TEZ oh mib

TRADE NAME(S):
Velcade

THERAPEUTIC CLASS:
Antineoplastic

GENERAL USES:
Multiple myeloma

DOSAGE FORMS:
Injection: 3.5 mg

BOSENTAN
boe SEN tan

TRADE NAME(S):
  Tracleer
THERAPEUTIC CLASS:
  Cardiac agent
GENERAL USES:
  Pulmonary hypertension
DOSAGE FORMS:
  Tablets: 62.5 mg, 125 mg

BOTULINUM TOXIN TYPE A
BOT yoo lin num TOKS in
TRADE NAME(S):
  Botox
THERAPEUTIC CLASS:
  Toxoid
GENERAL USES:
  Cervical dystonia, facial wrinkles, severe underarm sweating
DOSAGE FORMS:
  Injection: 100 units

BOTULINUM TOXIN TYPE B
BOT yoo lin num TOKS in
TRADE NAME(S):
  Myobloc
THERAPEUTIC CLASS:
  Toxoid
GENERAL USES:
  Cervical dystonia
DOSAGE FORMS:
  Injection: 2500 units, 5000 units, 10,000 units

BRIMONIDINE
bri MOE ni deen

TRADE NAME(S):
  Alphagan, Alphagan P
THERAPEUTIC CLASS:
  Ocular agent
GENERAL USES:
  Glaucoma/ocular hypertension
DOSAGE FORMS:
  Ophthalmic solution: 0.1%, 0.15%, 0.2%

BRIMONIDINE/ TIMOLOL
bri MOE ni deen/TYE moe lole
TRADE NAME(S):
  Combigan
THERAPEUTIC CLASS:
  Ocular agent
GENERAL USES:
  Glaucoma, ocular hypertension
DOSAGE FORMS:
  Ophthalmic solution: 0.2%/0.5%

BRINZOLAMIDE
brin ZOH la mide
TRADE NAME(S):
  Azopt
THERAPEUTIC CLASS:
  Ocular agent
GENERAL USES:
  Glaucoma/ocular hypertension
DOSAGE FORMS:
  Ophthalmic solution: 1%

BROMFENAC
BROME fen ak
TRADE NAME(S):
 Xibrom
THERAPEUTIC CLASS:
 Ocular agent
GENERAL USES:
 Postoperative cataract
 surgery
DOSAGE FORMS:
 Ophthalmic solution:
 0.09%

BROMOCRIPTINE
broe moe KRIP teen
TRADE NAME(S):
 Parlodel
THERAPEUTIC CLASS:
 Antiparkinson
 agent
GENERAL USES:
 Parkinson's
 disease
DOSAGE FORMS:
 Tablets: 2.5 mg;
 Capsules: 5 mg

BUDESONIDE
byoo DES oh nide
TRADE NAME(S):
 Entocort EC
THERAPEUTIC CLASS:
 Corticosteroid
GENERAL USES:
 Crohn's disease
DOSAGE FORMS:
 Capsules: 3 mg

BUDESONIDE (INHALED)
byoo DES oh nide
TRADE NAME(S):
 Pulmicort
THERAPEUTIC CLASS:
 Corticosteroid (inhaler)
GENERAL USES:
 Asthma (chronic)
DOSAGE FORMS:
 Inhaler: 200 mcg/
 inhalation; Inhalation
 suspension: 0.25 mg/
 2 mL, 0.5 mg/2 mL

BUDESONIDE (NASAL)
byoo DES oh nide
TRADE NAME(S):
 Rhinocort, Rhinocort Aqua
THERAPEUTIC CLASS:
 Corticosteroid (nasal)
GENERAL USES:
 Allergies
DOSAGE FORMS:
 Nasal aerosol: 32 mcg/
 spray

BUMETANIDE
byoo MET a nide
TRADE NAME(S):
 Bumex
THERAPEUTIC CLASS:
 Diuretic
GENERAL USES:
 CHF-related edema,
 hypertension
DOSAGE FORMS:
 Tablets: 0.5 mg, 1 mg,

2 mg; Injection: 0.5 mg,
1 mg, 2.5 mg

BUPRENORPHINE (SUBLINGUAL)
byoo pre NOR feen
TRADE NAME(S):
Subutex, Buprenex
THERAPEUTIC CLASS:
Analgesic (narcotic)
GENERAL USES:
Opioid dependence
DOSAGE FORMS:
Tablets, sublingual: 2 mg,
8 mg; Injection: 0.3 mg

BUPRENORPHINE/ NALOXONE (SUBLINGUAL)
byoo pre NOR feen/nal OKS one
TRADE NAME(S):
Suboxone
THERAPEUTIC CLASS:
Analgesic (narcotic)/
narcotic antagonist
GENERAL USES:
Opioid dependence
DOSAGE FORMS:
Tablets, sublingual: 2 mg/
0.5 mg, 8 mg/2 mg

BUPROPION
byoo PROE pee on
TRADE NAME(S):
Wellbutrin, Wellbutrin SR,
Wellbutrin XL, Budeprion
SR, Aplenzin
THERAPEUTIC CLASS:
Antidepressant
GENERAL USES:
Depression, seasonal
affective disorder
DOSAGE FORMS:
Tablets: 75 mg, 100 mg,
174 mg, 348 mg, 522 mg;
Sustained-release tablets:
100 mg, 150 mg, 200 mg;
Extended-release tablets:
150 mg, 300 mg

BUPROPION
byoo PROE pee on
TRADE NAME(S):
Zyban, Buproban
THERAPEUTIC CLASS:
Smoking deterrent
GENERAL USES:
Smoking cessation
DOSAGE FORMS:
Sustained-release tablets:
150 mg

BUSPIRONE
byoo SPYE rone
TRADE NAME(S):
BuSpar
THERAPEUTIC CLASS:
Antianxiety agent
GENERAL USES:
Depression
DOSAGE FORMS:
Tablets: 5 mg, 10 mg,
15 mg, 30 mg

BUTABARBITAL
byoo ta BAR bi tal
TRADE NAME(S):
  Butisol
THERAPEUTIC CLASS:
  Sedative/hypnotic
GENERAL USES:
  Insomnia (short-term therapy)
DOSAGE FORMS:
  Tablets: 15 mg, 30 mg, 50 mg, 100 mg; Elixir: 30 mg/5 mL

BUTENAFINE
byoo TEN a feen
TRADE NAME(S):
  Mentax
THERAPEUTIC CLASS:
  Antifungal (topical)
GENERAL USES:
  Athlete's foot
DOSAGE FORMS:
  Cream: 1%

CABERGOLINE
ca BER goe leen
TRADE NAME(S):
  Dostinex
THERAPEUTIC CLASS:
  Dopamine receptor agonist
GENERAL USES:
  Hyperprolactinemia
DOSAGE FORMS:
  Tablets: 0.5 mg

CALCIPOTRIENE
kal si POE try een
TRADE NAME(S):
  Dovonex
THERAPEUTIC CLASS:
  Antipsoriatic (topical)
GENERAL USES:
  Psoriasis
DOSAGE FORMS:
  Ointment, Solution, and Cream: 0.005%

CALCIPOTRIENE/ BETAMETHASONE DIPROPIONATE
kal si POE try een/bay ta METH a sone
TRADE NAME(S):
  Taclonex
THERAPEUTIC CLASS:
  Dermatological agent
GENERAL USES:
  Psoriasis
DOSAGE FORMS:
  Ointment and Topical suspension: 0.005%/0.064%

CALCITONIN
kal si TOE nin
TRADE NAME(S):
  Miacalcin
THERAPEUTIC CLASS:
  Hormone
GENERAL USES:
  Osteoporosis, Paget's disease

DOSAGE FORMS:
Injection:
400 international
units; Nasal spray:
200 international units/
actuation

CALCITONIN-SALMON (rDNA ORIGIN)
kal si TOE nin
TRADE NAME(S):
Fortical
THERAPEUTIC CLASS:
Hormone
GENERAL USES:
Postmenopausal
osteoporosis
DOSAGE FORMS:
Nasal spray:
200 international units/
actuation

CALCIUM CHLORIDE
KAL see um KLOR ide
TRADE NAME(S):
Calcium Chloride
THERAPEUTIC CLASS:
Electrolyte
GENERAL USES:
Replacement
DOSAGE FORMS:
Injection: 10%

CALCIUM GLUCONATE
KAL see um GLOO koe nate
TRADE NAME(S):
Calcium Gluconate

THERAPEUTIC CLASS:
Electrolyte
GENERAL USES:
Replacement
DOSAGE FORMS:
Injection: 10%

CANDESARTAN
kan de SAR tan
TRADE NAME(S):
Atacand
THERAPEUTIC CLASS:
Antihypertensive
GENERAL USES:
Hypertension, CHF
DOSAGE FORMS:
Tablets: 4 mg, 8 mg,
16 mg, 32 mg

CAPECITABINE
ka pe SITE a been
TRADE NAME(S):
Xeloda
THERAPEUTIC CLASS:
Antineoplastic
GENERAL USES:
Metastatic breast
cancer
DOSAGE FORMS:
Tablets: 150 mg,
500 mg

CAPTOPRIL
KAP toe pril
TRADE NAME(S):
Capoten
THERAPEUTIC CLASS:
Antihypertensive,
cardiac agent